Praise for Pixie Dust:

Pixie Dust is a treasure trove of illuminating jewels of wisdom and practical advice from an obviously experienced and enlightened young mother. It emanates a loving and common sense approach to the difficult and often frustrating endeavor of new motherhood, giving comfort in the realm of the unknown. A most enjoyable read and highly recommended.

—Lynda Henry, R.N.CM

I read this book prior to my first and second child. It helped me physically prepare for them but mentally grasp what to expect! As a dietitian and a lactation consultant I felt that I knew it all. Loralyn was able to make this book personal enough that I actually realized it's a baby I'm having not a science project! She helps you learn to be a good caretaker, nurturer, and provider but mostly a great mom! You will love her humor in reading this book and greatly appreciate her detailed tidbits! I passed my copy of the book around to all of my friends expecting and will recommend it to everyone I know.

—Keri Hale, RD/LD, IBCLC

pixie dust

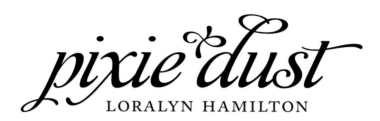

pixie dust

LORALYN HAMILTON

*magical insights for childbirth
and life with little one*

TATE PUBLISHING & *Enterprises*

Published by Tate Publishing & Enterprises, LLC
127 E. Trade Center Terrace | Mustang, Oklahoma 73064 USA
1.888.361.9473 | www.tatepublishing.com

Tate Publishing is committed to excellence in the publishing industry. The company reflects the philosophy established by the founders, based on Psalm 68:11,
"The Lord gave the word and great was the company of those who published it."

Book design copyright © 2009 by Tate Publishing, LLC. All rights reserved.
Illustrated by Diane Haxel
Cover design by Amber Gulilat
Interior design by Jeff Fisher

Published in the United States of America

ISBN: 978-1-61566-267-8
1. Health & Fitness, Pregnancy & Childbirth
2. Family & Relationships, Parenting, Motherhood
09.12.08

Dear Friend ~

As parenthood draws near, you may find that there are many things that either the books haven't told you or you've completely forgotten; things you wish you had known beforehand that would have saved so much time and frustration. You may find yourself wishing for a magical helper, perhaps some *Pixie Dust*, to offer unique and helpful insights that make childbirth and life with Baby just a little easier. That helper has finally arrived!

This book is filled with advice from my own experience as well as wonderful wisdom from other mothers, and helps to bridge the confusing and overwhelming gap between the last months of pregnancy to early life with Baby. Throughout the book you will see selections called *Pixie Dust.* Sprinkle these magical insights over the many tasks surrounding childbirth and the days to follow, and you are sure to find that even the smallest piece of advice can provide priceless comfort and peace of mind. Our gift is hindsight, gathered here, to help pave your way to a sweeter, simpler tomorrow. Now you can spend *your* time envisioning and creating a more peaceful and joyful life with little one!

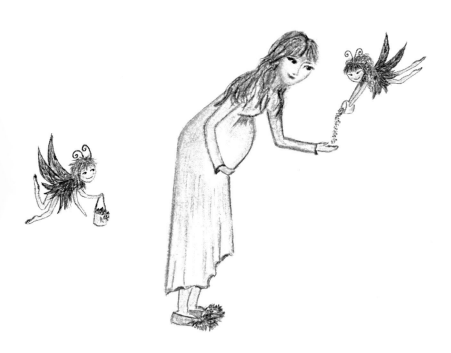

"All you need is faith, trust
     and a little bit of *Pixie Dust*!"

—Peter Pan

Dedications

This book is dedicated to my daughter, Caelyn Diane. Without the blessed experience of her birth and life, none of this would have come to pass. And to Daniel, my Superman, by my side learning, laughing, and loving through it all.

To my Momma ... where are the words?

Because of you, I am.

Acknowledgments

A heartfelt Thank You to Jennifer, Kelly M., Valorie, Kelly H., Keri, Tara, Emily, and Suzanne. This book began with you in mind and has ended with you within. Thank you for your loving support, advice, and most importantly, your friendship.

A special recognition to my daddy, my hero: you have always inspired me to be true to myself and encouraged me to pursue my dreams without exception.

To my brother Russ, "Half of me breathes in you … thoughts of love remain true … " Nixons band.

Thank you to my grandparents and my extended family, all of whom have been a source of inspiration, encouragement, and unconditional love throughout my life.

Thank you to Lansinoh®, Dr. Brown's Bottles, and Boppy for allowing your products to be featured within this book. A special thank you to Gina from Lansinoh®. Your assistance and encouragement has been a blessing.

Thank you to everyone at Tate Publishing who has helped to make this lifelong dream come true: Stacy, Rachael, Dave, Katie, Amber, Jeff, and Dr. Tate. Your guidance has brought to life the voice and spirit of this work.

Morning Prayer

Now I wake up from my sleep
I pray the Lord my soul to keep
Love and guard me through the day
And help me bless along the way.
Amen

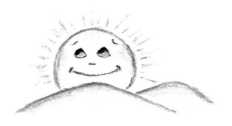

Getting Ready For Baby!

Clean the house, tidy up yourself, purchase necessities, get the nursery ready, pack Baby's diaper bag, pack your bag, make your call list, prepare and make arrangements for siblings, discuss birthing plans, and ... relax!

Nesting

Everything goes! Dust bunnies under the couch will see their last days (at least for a while!). The junk closet begins to catapult unnecessary items every time you open its door. The "spare" bedroom (now the nursery) becomes filled with boxes and gifts from baby showers that demand to be organized or else burst out into the hall. You say with an inner cringe, "I'll do that tomorrow." Well, congratulations! Your need for organization has thrown you into what is now "tomorrow" and you are successfully within the "nesting" phase ... out with the old, in with the new!

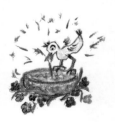

Tidy Up!

Shave the bikini line and trim the bush!
Heaven forbid they have to
break out the buzz saw!
Get a pedicure—a spa pedicure!
You can't even see your toes
much less reach them.
A pedicure will de-crustify the
heels, paint the nails,
and massage your poor, tired
stalks. Well worth the money!
And your nurses and doctors
will thank you!

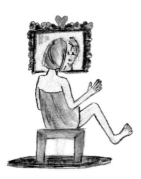

Hospital Necessities for Baby

Pack this now! Include in the diaper bag to take to the hospital:

- Going Home Outfit
- Diapers and Wipes
- Diaper Rash Ointment
- Pacifiers (sterilized)
- Nail File
- Nasal Aspirator
- Receiving Blankets
- Bottles (sterilized)
- Gas Drops
- Burp Cloths
- Disposable Diaper Bags
- Hats and Socks

pixie dust

At the end of this book you will find comprehensive lists of most everything you will need before, during and after Baby's arrival. It might be helpful to take these lists with you as you register or complete your Baby and Mommy necessity purchases.

Hospital Necessities for Mommy

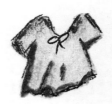

- Robe
- Slippers
- PJs or Gown
- Pillows (colored cases)
- Hair Clip or Rubber Band
- Lotion and Body Spray
- Toiletries to Shower
- Lip Balm and Make Up
- Going Home Outfit
- Paper and Pen
- Nursing Bras, Pads, and Breast Cream
- Spouse, Coach, or Friend
- Music for Labor
- Music Player

pixie dust

Life brings about many circumstances that are out of our control. For whatever reason, having a spouse around during labor and delivery may not always be possible. It's a good idea to designate a "go to" person if a spouse or coach is not going to be able to be with you during labor and delivery. Even with a spouse or coach, you may need additional help, so choose someone who can be with you if needed, and can run errands just after Baby is born should you need something the hospital doesn't provide (like good food, for instance!).

Hospital Necessities for Spouse or Coach

- Snacks and Quarters–For vending machines, the cafeteria closes at night.

- Sweatshirt–It may be cold in the hospital room.

- Camera, Camcorder, & Batteries–Make sure they know how to use these properly.

- Cell Phone & Call List–Designate this person to let family/friends know about Baby.

Note to Spouse, Coach or Friend

If you are a spouse, it's a good idea to take some responsibility for a few things before Baby arrives, like installing the car seat, putting together baby furniture, and helping to keep the house clean. Although you are excited, this can be a scary time for Mommy. During labor and delivery, there are many things you can do to help comfort her like rub her neck and back, feed her ice chips, use a wet washcloth to cool her down, and hold her hand to give her reassurance that you are there to help. It's important to remember to keep your cool and be patient, as her emotions will be swinging like crazy!

Note to Mommy

If you have a spouse, remember to include them in this process. This is their life and little one too. Allow them to step up and help with things before Baby arrives. Let them put together furniture and take care of assembling/installing car seats, strollers, and toys. During the last few months of pregnancy, physical activity can induce Premature Labor and Baby needs all the time it can get to mature inside you, so let others do the work.

After delivery, let your spouse change the diapers, feed Baby (if you're not nursing full-time), and spend time alone with little one so that they too, may bond with Baby. Things won't always get done the way you would do them and that's okay, you need all the help you can get. If there is something that needs to be done differently, approach it from a "we" stand point, not a "you" so that you don't appear to be criticizing. After all, you are both learning. As long as Baby isn't in harm's way, just let go and enjoy this time with your spouse and your new little one, there will never be another experience like it!

Necessities for the Nursery

- Crib / Bassinet
- Diaper Pail / Bags
- Clothes
- Bedding / Sheets
- Diapers / Wipes
- Dresser
- Receiving Blankets
- Baskets / Hangers
- Boppy
- Sleep Positioner
- Wipe Warmer
- Detergent
- Changing Table
- Bottle Warmer
- Medicines
- Carrier / Sling
- Bath Items
- Monitor
- Swing / Bouncer
- Feeding Items
- Hamper
- Safe Cleaning Spray
- Stain Remover
- Totes
- Play Mats
- Hot Water Pads
- Rocker

Necessities for Home and Travel

- Car Seat / Travel System
- Diaper Bag
- Baby Wash / Shampoo / Lotion
- Finger Nail File
- Bottles / Nipples / Liners
- Finger Nail Clippers
- Colic Tablets / Acetaminophen
- Nasal Aspirator
- Diaper Rash Ointment
- Gas Drops / Teething Gel
- Baskets for Dishwasher (2)
- Scrub Brush
- Small & Large Washcloths
- Bottle Brushes
- Disposable Diaper Bags
- Clothes
- Wipe Holder for Diaper Bag
- Pacifiers

Car Seats

Did anyone tell you that you can't leave the hospital with your baby without a car seat properly installed? Did anyone tell you that car seats are not as easy to install as one might think? Did anyone tell you that some car seats will not fit correctly in your car? Did anyone tell you that the type of car seat you buy does make a difference? Did anyone tell you your newborn will not fit nicely inside the car seat? Well, now someone has! Research the safest seat, have it installed by a local fire station, take a safety course, read the instructions, and get some pillows or receiving blankets to fit around Baby's body while in the seat.

pixie dust

Extra car seat bases (a base is what holds the carrier, which is also the car seat for babies) are nice to have for additional cars. You might even get one for grandparents or caregivers who might be toting little one around.

Travel Systems

Strollers that have it all: car seat/carrier, car seat base, a carry all basket, cup holders, and of course a snack tray—the latter two not to be used until Baby is much older. These are wonderful! Just be sure to look for one that is stable, easy to maneuver, easy to fold up and down, and light enough to lift with one hand. Baby will often be in the other!

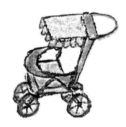

Bassinets

A bedside bassinet is a must have for the first few months! Rocking and vibrating features are well worth the investment and some even have soothing sounds and music. Being able to swing your arm up over the side of the bassinet to comfort Baby at 3:00 a.m. is worth its weight in gold. Just be sure to wash all bedding before bringing Baby home.

Since babies are supposed to be put to sleep on their backs, sleep positioners are also a must have to keep Baby from rolling over. Just be sure to give Baby plenty of tummy time during the day to exercise (and prevent bald spots!).

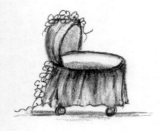

pixie dust

Little newbies are so tiny and so still when they sleep, you will wonder if they are really breathing! Keep a little flashlight by the bed at night to check on Baby or to find pacifiers when they go missing.

Pacifiers

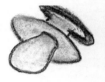

Plug it up! Although some believe that pacifiers have caused problems with orthodontia growth and speech ability if used during later toddler years, they serve so many functions it is hard not to promote their use. They comfort Baby, they give you much needed quiet time, and they give Baby something else to suck on instead of using you as a pacifier. Even the American Academy of Pediatrics recommends that babies take pacifiers during the first year of life as they are supposed to help reduce the risk of SIDS.

If you want Baby to use them, wash them (sterilize) and take them to the hospital with you and ask the nurses to use them. If you do not want Baby to take a pacifier, be sure to let the staff know beforehand— the hospital will probably have you sign a release either way.

pixie dust

If Baby is picky, try different nipple shapes—one will eventually work!

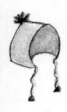

Baby Clothes

Unless you give birth to a child by the name of Big Ben or Boxy Bertha, your baby will be a lot smaller than what you imagined. Most newborn and 0–3 month outfits will be big on Baby for the first several weeks. You might want to buy a few cheap preemie outfits just in case.

The main items you will need for coming home and the first few weeks are: a going home outfit, sleepers, long-sleeved front snap shirts (with cuff sleeves so you can turn them over Baby's hands when nails are long), hats (help to maintain body temperature), socks (make sure they don't bind Baby's ankles), pants, and gowns.

Pants are nice for car rides—it's easier to buckle them in. Gowns are nice for nighttime—you don't have to mess with snaps when you're changing a diaper in the dark half asleep!

pixie dust

Buy a soft nightlight for the nursery to use for midnight diaper changes.

Yes, there really is a Dryer Monster. And yes, it will eat little socks. Buy a hosiery bag to wash socks and bibs. But don't wash them together as the Velcro on the bibs sticks to everything!

Does it really matter what kind of detergent you wash Baby's clothes in? No, not unless you notice that Baby has a rash of some sort—then you might want to consider a change (or unless sensitive skin runs in your family). However, stain remover is a *must!* In fact, buy several bottles—put one by the changing table, one by the washer, and one in the kitchen.

Oh No! No Leaky Diaper Here!

If someone told you to start buying diapers every time you went to the grocery store, hopefully you listened! Just be sure to buy bigger sizes too so you don't stock up on all one size. At first, Baby will go through eight to ten diapers a day. You will freak out the first time you need to change a diaper and there aren't any to be found! Of the parents consulted, most agree that Pampers are better than others and Pampers Swaddlers really are softer than most diapers. Once Baby gets a little bigger, try Pampers Flex with Baby Dry. These really do stop the leaks!

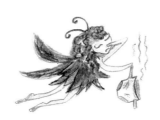

pixie dust

Once the diapers begin to fit "just right,"
it's time to move up to the next stage. This
will help to avoid leaks and blowouts.

If your baby could talk, you'd probably hear a few curse words when applying a cold wipe to Baby's bare bottom. Buy a wipe warmer. Oh, and thicker wipes seem to work better at cleaning up "thicker" messes.

There are a lot of different diaper rash ointments; you may have to try a few to see what works for you. Lansinoh® makes a great diaper rash ointment, which is designed to include the benefits of a white ointment (zinc oxide) that rubs in clear. This product is fragrance free and non-comedogenic.

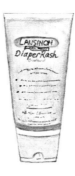

pixie dust

As a rule, breastfed babies have less diaper rash than babies who are formula fed, so if your breastfed baby has diaper rash, take a look at what you've been eating that might be the culprit (tomatoes, alcohol, peppers, etc.). More about this later!

Accessorize!

Welcome to parenthood! Here you will become familiar with an entirely different meaning of the word "accessorize!"

The Snot Bulb... another *must have,* also known as the nasal aspirator. Keep one in the car and one in the house in case Baby spits up and begins to choke. Remember to suction mouth before nose (M before N). These are also good for little boogies. Just be sure to buy the ones with the tapered end and an opening for easy cleaning so something doesn't come to life inside it!

Either buy a few lap pads (they come in a pack of three), or be prepared to continue in a perpetual state of laundry as changing messy diapers can become messy everything! Your diaper bag may come with a washable changing pad to use as well.

pixie dust

To keep costs down, cut several little pieces of cloth (they can even match your nursery) just the size of Baby and use these over the changing table cover when changing diapers.

Icky tummies are sometimes difficult to diagnose, much less treat. If you have a hot water pad or bottle, you can fill it with warm water and place on Baby's tummy to relieve discomfort. You can also use it to warm up Baby's bed so the covers aren't cold when you lay them down. Just be sure to remove the bottle before laying Baby down.

Day One: Home with Baby … arm asleep for the umpteenth time … the phone keeps ringing and between Baby, the blanket, the bottle (or boob), the pacifier, not being able to scratch the reoccurring itch on my nose, and my sanity, I swear I'm going to be forced by evolution to quickly sprout another pair of hands! Why haven't they invented something to help me? Where is everyone when I need them? Am I too old to scream, "I want my MOMMMMYYYYY!"

Well, rest easy (or easier)…buy a Boppy! This little donut shaped pillow fits around you and holds Baby to you while you do what you need to do…at least while you're sitting.

But if you've got to be on the go—buy a sling! Babies love them because they remind them of the womb…dark and cozy and right next to mom.

Instant baby sitter you ask? Portable bouncers or swings are wonderful! You can carry them from room to room (nice if you want to take a shower) and take them places outside the home.

pixie dust

Buy a lot of batteries! Things like swings and toys to entertain run on batteries and they run out rather quickly so stock up.

You never know whose little snot covered fingers or mouth may have touched the toy you just bought from the store for your baby (or has been given to Baby by a friend). Since you cannot immerse most baby toys and rattles in water, safe cleaning spray is great for just this. Also use this on highchairs and any other surfaces Baby may touch.

I'm sure you've heard that baby powder is not recommended for use on a consistent basis for respiratory reasons. However, it's really nice to have around when there's no time for a bath and Baby's just had a really messy diaper!

pixie dust

Sprinkle baby powder in diaper pails to eliminate odors. It works every time and it helps the pail to work more smoothly!

Necessities for Mommy After Birth

- Extra Large Sanitary Napkins–You will have a massive period for several days.

- Nursing Bras–If you are nursing, your breasts will be even bigger once your milk comes in!

- Breast Cream–If you are nursing, this will help heal sore skin on and around the nipples.

- Nursing Pads for Bra–Even if you're not nursing, these will help contain milk until it dries up.

- Anti-Bacterial Wipes–To help keep yours and "well-meaning" baby holder's hands clean.

- Ibuprofen–Helps with pain and inflammation.

- Diaper Bag–This will become your purse, so find a cute one!

- Journal–For two reasons: to track what you've eaten if you're nursing, and to write down your thoughts and things that made your own life easier during this time. Makes a good keep sake!

- Girdle Panties...

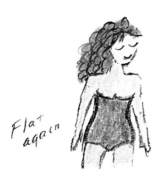

Flat again

pixie dust

Whether you've had a vaginal birth or a cesarean, buy girdle panties to help hold in and re-train tummy muscles while they are healing. They will help flatten your tummy and will keep muscles from aching as much. These will also keep pants from rubbing up against cesarean stitches/scars.

How Could I Ever Love Another As Much?

Feeling a little guilt and a lot of anxiety over how your first child will accept your second or third or fourth? If you're like most of us, you're already putting yourself in their shoes… imagining how scary it must feel to know "something" is about to change your life as you know it. So you struggle with issues like jealousy and how your child will react to the decrease in attention from you, or how you could ever love another as much… all very valid and very common emotional issues. In fact, I don't know a mom who hasn't struggled with these concerns.

Here are a few things to help you feel a little more at peace with everyone's new adjustment period.

Try to spend a little bit of quality time with your child every day—even if it's just five minutes of your undivided attention—to remind them of who they are to you and how very much you love them. "Try" being the operative word as there will be days that have run into nights that have run into days. You may be consumed and you will be tired. Just find peace in the fact that you and your children will all be okay. You'll get back on track and everyone will adjust to the added blessings of your new little bundle of joy.

Include your child in the entire process, from decorating the nursery to taking pictures after Baby is born. Buy a dolly and show your child how to feed it and hold it and praise your child for what a big help they are!

When Baby arrives, help your child feel connected to Baby by giving your child a present from Baby. Tell them it's a "thank you" for helping to take care of Baby.

There are a few technical issues you may need to work out for your child before Baby arrives. Here are a few things you need to consider and be prepared for in order to make the transition go smoothly for your family.

Some parents want their children to be a part of the birthing process; others feel it might be too dramatic. Either way, you need to make arrangements for a designated caretaker for your child during and after the birthing process.

Pack a bag of clothes, toys, and familiar things, so your child will feel comfortable. If your child is to stay the night somewhere unfamiliar, you might even do a trial run and let your child stay the night with the chosen caregiver before Baby's arrival to acclimate your child to new surroundings.

pixie dust

Don't forget to give authorization to your childs' school as to who will be picking up your child!

Mommy's Little Piggy

Can't anything be easy? You'd think that feeding Baby would be the most natural and easiest of tasks. After all, you don't think twice about your innate ability to stuff your face! However, whether you breastfeed or bottle feed, you may encounter things like how long can breast milk sit out before it spoils, what products really are helpful to have, and where to find helpful tips and encouragement should this become a daunting task. Here you'll find a few answers that may help you along the way!

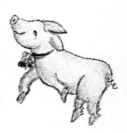

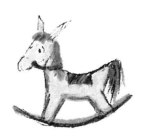

Upon My High Horse. . .

While breastfeeding is a personal choice, keep in mind that you are making a choice that affects not only you but also Baby. I don't need to tell you that breast milk is best—you hear it everywhere. The American Academy of Pediatrics states that breast milk reduces the risk of infection due to colds and viruses by increasing Baby's immunities. Studies have also shown that babies who are breastfed have slightly higher IQ's. And babies who are breastfed grow naturally as opposed to formula fed babies who may gain too much weight and may be more prone to childhood obesity. Well, that's all well and good for Baby, but what's in it for you, you ask? Well, read on!

There's no doubt that you will have a little (or a lot) of weight to take off after Baby arrives. Breastfeeding will help you to burn up to 500 extra calories a day making it easier to shed that pregnancy weight!

Breastfeeding is *much* cheaper than formula and you don't have to wash all those bottles and nipples all the time, nor do you have to worry about leaving the house with a bottle and formula (unless you're leaving Baby with a caretaker). In fact, breastfeeding, in and of itself, is virtually free, whereas formula can cost over $150 a month!

So let's do the math. Depending on the brand and your baby's needs, a can of formula can cost anywhere from $14.99 and up (way up). If we take the cheapest we can buy at around $14.99, which makes 85 ounces of formula, and divide this by 30 ounces (the average of what a baby will eat in a day, and this will vary depending on

Baby's age), then you can see that one can will feed Baby for around 3 days. If 31 days in a month divided by 3 is roughly 10, you will have to buy 10 cans of cheap formula in any given month. So what is 10 X $14.99? $149.90 and we haven't even included tax. I don't know about you but I can think of many a things I could use that money on when Baby can get the best milk for free. Momma needs a new pair of shoes!

If you decide you would like to alternate between breastfeeding and bottle feeding, there are a few precautions of which to be aware. First, unless you are pumping or nursing on a consistent schedule, you run the risk of depleting your breast milk supply. Your breasts produce milk according to demand, the more it's needed, the more it's produced. The less it's needed, the less it's produced. In fact, even if you've chosen to breastfeed exclusively and Baby begins to sleep through the night, you may find that not nursing during the nighttime hours causes your milk production to lessen.

A second precaution is that when alternating breast milk and formula, you might not be able to pinpoint the culprit of an upset tummy and Baby's digestive system will be very sensitive during the first several months. It will take more effort on your part but then there are some upsides to alternating too. Someone else can feed Baby when you can't, and you just might not feel like a milk cow in the process!

For most of us, exclusive breastfeeding will delay the return of your menstrual cycle. This does *not* mean that you cannot get pregnant during this time. You can, so if you don't want another bambino on the way, use precautions!

Breastfeeding causes the uterus to contract, which helps it to return to normal size more quickly. Breastfeeding also has health benefits including reduced post partum depression, reduced risks for ovarian and breast cancers and osteoporosis.

And the bonding process is amazing! Never again will you feel closer to anything on earth. Need I say more?

pixie dust:

If you decide not to nurse, or when it comes time to wean Baby, ask your lactation consultant or your doctor for tips on how to do this gently for both your sake and Baby's. Just know that when you feel it's time to wean Baby, this process can be a hormonally challenging one for you as well.

Breastfeeding Accessories?

If you're breastfeeding, do you really need any accessories? Well, yes and no. Technically you can get along just fine without any of these, but most of these sure make things a whole lot easier!

Before going into all the handy items you can use for breastfeeding, I would like to give a shout out to Lansinoh®. This company's *sole* purpose is to assist mothers with the breastfeeding process. They provide just about everything you need from breast pumps and accessories to helpful tips and encouraging words on the breastfeeding process. All Lansinoh® Brand breastfeeding products are highly recommended by moms and breastfeeding educators.

Your nipples will have a *slight* adjustment period at the beginning of the breastfeeding process. Use Lansinoh HPA® Lanolin, the world's safest and purest lanolin. This *really* will help soothe your nipples.

pixie dust

If you find that your nipples are extremely sore during this adjustment period, be careful of what you use to wash this area. Harsh soaps (sometimes using any soap at all) can be over drying causing the nipples and skin to be more chaffed than necessary.

Lansinoh® Breast Milk Storage Bags are wonderful to store your pumped breast milk... easy to write on (date of milk pumped) and easy to seal!

Lansinoh ®has also developed a product called LatchAssist™, a simple tool designed to gently draw out temporarily flattened or inverted nipples due to milk engorgement or swelling in the early days after birth.

First of all, couldn't someone come up with a better word than "engorged" to describe what happens when our breasts overflow with milk? I mean, as if our body and its processes don't already have enough hideous words associated with them! I looked up a synonym in the thesaurus but found words like puffy and bloated... none of which more positively described this rather negative experience. What about "her breasts were replete with milk"? Hmmm ... sounds like something out of an explicit romance novel. Either way, this is just one of the reasons you will want to have a breast pump on hand. However, if you are in pain, it is recommended that you use a hot pack to relieve the pain and then hand express milk by gently massaging the breast tissue.

pixie dust

It's nice to have a supply of milk on hand in case you want to leave Baby with a caretaker or in case you need to take medicine that you don't want to expose to Baby.

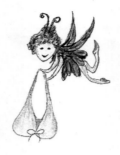

Wearing a bra twenty-four hours a day will help prevent and resolve several issues. Consistently wearing a bra will keep your nipples and breasts from becoming sore, it will keep you from leaking all over the place, and it will help to prevent the dreaded "sagging" after Baby is completely done with nursing. Just purchase a loosely fitting sports bra to wear at night and either a nursing bra or your regular bra in larger sizes for during the day.

pixie dust

When purchasing a nursing bra or a bra to wear post pregnancy, slide your hand inside the bra and cup your hand over your breast while fitting the bra to you. This should be close to the size you will be once your milk comes in.

You will find that lots of things will leak over the next few months...diapers, bottles, and yes, your boobs (when they are "replete" with milk!). This is one of the many functions that nursing pads serve. You may not need these often once Baby is on a good nursing schedule, but they are very nice to have in the beginning. Cotton washable nursing pads allow your skin to breathe, which reduces additional aggravation to your nipples. Lansinoh® makes wonderful washable nursing pads as well as disposables to take in the diaper bag!

pixie dust

Nursing pads are also nice to use as, should I dare say it...falsies! When you nurse, one breast may have a tendency to be bigger than the other (especially if Baby nurses for the most part from one side— which is very common) and two or three pads fit perfectly in your bra to help even out the difference.

Mother's Milk ...

Here are a few notes about breast milk in general, things like how to store it, what to store it in and how long it will stay fresh once stored.

Aaaahhhh ... "liquid gold!", also known as colostrum. This is the fluid that comes in just before your breast milk and is known for its amazing healthful properties to newborn babies. Did you know that people actually pump this (as well as breast milk) and sell it! Mothers who want their babies to have its benefits but can't nurse, can buy colostrum and breast milk from a Milk Bank.

Does breast milk have an expiration date like regular milk? Yep! Follow the Rule of 5: five hours at room temperature, five days in the fridge, five months in the freezer (or 6–12 months in deep freezer). If you are storing breast milk, be sure to write the date and time on the bag so you know which bag to use first.

pixie dust

Breast milk has healing properties especially on yours and Baby's skin. If your nipples become sore, let a little breast milk dry on them to help them heal. If Baby has a nursing rash around the mouth, let a little breast milk dry on the area to help clear up the rash. You can also put a drop in eyes to heal conjunctivitis.

There will come a point during breastfeeding when you wonder if something you ate may have upset Baby's tummy. Days will have run into nights and you will have lost all track of time as to when you ate what. If you can, keep a journal of everything you eat so that you can determine immediately what might cause Baby to have gas or discomfort. Anything that makes you gassy will probably make Baby gassy too. But more often than not, things will bother Baby that won't bother you. Broccoli, caffeine, chocolate, onions, spices, sugar, eggs, and any kind of dairy are just a few examples.

pixie dust

Caffeine has a tendency to build up in Baby's system—they don't process it like we do. It's hidden in things like cool whip, chocolate, teas, and sodas. So you may want to opt for decaf but always go for the chocolate!

For some of you, breastfeeding will be a piece of cake! Mmmm ... cake! For others, getting Baby to latch on, getting a good milk supply, getting Baby to feed without falling asleep, or being able to determine what you've eaten that's upsetting Baby's tummy may seem discouraging.

Be sure to keep the card from your lactation consultants at the hospital. Don't hesitate to call if you have any questions regarding the breastfeeding process (like what medicines are okay for you to take while breastfeeding). For instance, antihistamines for colds or allergies are okay if taken sparingly; they have no ill effect on Baby other than maybe some drowsiness, but they can dry up your milk if you take too much too often. Call just to be sure!

But now it's 3:00 a.m ... Baby is crying, you're tired, you've tried everything you know to try to get Baby to eat and to soothe Baby. You yourself want your mommy, but it's really too late to call. So what do we moms do when we have no outside adult contact with the rest of the world? We jump online … "maybe, just maybe someone will have some encouraging words to help me through the night." And someone usually does. There are a lot of different forums out there for moms–Kellymom and Mamasource to name a couple. Lansinoh® also offers Nurture Notes, which contains helpful breastfeeding hints, facts, and encouraging words at www.lansinoh.com. You can also visit a new online community by Lansinoh® at www.lansinohmoms.com. Don't be afraid to get out there and ask questions!

We are out there, you are *not* alone.

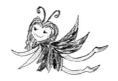

To Drink or Not to Drink...

That really is a good question! Sometimes it's just nice to know you have options. The La Leche League (the foundation for women who breastfeed), says to nurse only after the effects of the alcohol have worn off. The alcohol has been processed by your kidneys and is out of your system and therefore, out of your breast milk. Some doctors say to "pump and dump" so that Baby doesn't get any of the alcohol— just as a precaution. Ask your doctor or pediatrician what they recommend.

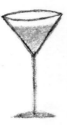

pixie dust

Just remember that when two or three glasses of wine caught a nice buzz back in the day, now one glass will send you three sheets to the wind!

Stay Organized

Early morning sunrise…and you're wondering where on earth you put the most recently used bottle, knowing full well you have to clean it, prepare the formula or milk, and change a diaper all before Baby's crying escalates into a full blown tantrum, waking the entire household. It's frustrating times like this that make you realize you need one "spot" for everything. So, whether you're nursing or bottle feeding, you will want to set up a little station in your kitchen with a drying rack for bottles, nipples, pump bottles, and other accessories.

pixie dust

Yes, we are all lazy during nighttime feedings. Some of us are lazy all the time ... I mean, it's not like we have anything to do—at all! Help yourself with cleaning ... buy a little tote that sits in the sink. Fill it with hot, soapy water so that you can toss in bottles and nipples when dirty. It's wonderful to come back to a cleanly soaked bottle and nipple; it's like a little fairy did it!

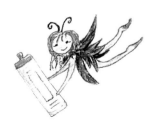

Bottle Feeding

Lions and Tigers and Bears, Oh My! Here is where you become overwhelmed with what products to buy. What bottles work best, what formula to use, the nipples, the burp cloths, and even the water! Recommendations are coming at you from all ends, but what really works?

Well, a lot of this will be trial and error to determine yours and Baby's preferences. Even if you breastfeed, you may want to explore the option of giving Baby a bottle of breast milk or formula. It's just nice to know what other mothers have found to be really helpful in resolving certain issues, and a few things that were not so helpful as well.

It's amazing the things they come up with to help cultivate our "laziness!" (As if taking care of a newborn could be even anywhere in the vicinity of laziness—no matter the short cuts you take!) If you bottle feed but don't like having to clean 100 bottles a day (I'd like to meet the person who describes one of their spare time interests as cleaning bottles) then use bottles with disposable liners for breast milk or formula. Playtex Nursers® are wonderful! The liners also help with gas and tummy issues (Baby's, not yours—though if you're having trouble too, you might *try* the infant gas drops!).

Peas, Porridge, Hot? Baby may prefer warm milk as opposed to cold. If you use regular bottles, you may want a bottle warmer. You can place these at bedside at nighttime. Prepare the bottles before you go to bed, so you don't have to mess with making them in the middle of the night. But if you're using liners, you'll have to warm up the milk by placing the bottle in a cup under warm running water from the faucet. Check the temperature by dabbing a little milk on your wrist before giving it to baby. If you can feel it, it's too hot!

Baby got gas! (The new nursery time Rap Song!) If Baby has a lot of trouble with gas and tummy problems, Dr. Brown's® bottles are highly recommended. These bottles are patented with a vacuum-free, positive flow feeding system, which helps to eliminate the ingestion of air (causing gas and upset stomach) during feedings. These will take a little extra effort to clean and are a little more expensive, but if Baby really has tummy problems, it's worth it.

Do you like the smell of burnt rubber? Chances are neither will Baby. Buy silicon nipples. If you buy other nipples (usually the brown ones) and boil them, they will smell like rubber and they don't last as long anyway.

pixie dust

Nipples are labeled according to the months in which babies need that particular size. These labels are as follows: slow (usually for the first few months), medium, or fast. If Baby seems frustrated with the slow, move to the medium.

Choosing a formula will *definitely* be trial and error at first. There is formula available for babies who are prone to reflux or gastrological discomforts, but these are more expensive. Unless Baby has reflux or other tummy issues, try the less expensive ones first. It's important to pick a formula and try to stick with it, so Baby has a chance to adjust to it. Don't switch back and forth if you can avoid it.

Purchase a formula holder (usually holds four servings of formula) to use when going out. This way you have measured servings ready to pour into a bottle when Baby is hungry.

It is recommended that you use nursery or bottled water when bottle feeding so that Baby doesn't receive impurities from tap water. These days you never really know what you're getting, but at least you can say you tried!

Baby will spit up and it would be nice if it didn't always have to happen on your shirt! Use burp cloths to burp Baby during and after feeding. You can also place these under Baby's chin if Baby's mouth has a tendency to leak while feeding.

Oh Boy (Or Girl!) Here We Go!

You're sitting there daydreaming about how it's going to go ... you have everything laid out just the way you want, bags packed, nursery done, call list made. You've even read all the great books like *What to Expect When You're Expecting* and *The GirlFriend's Guide to Pregnancy,* but there is something lingering in the back of your mind ... "what don't I know?" Here are a few more things you might not know about Eating and Delivery, Inductions, Vaginal Births, C-Sections, and Recovery.

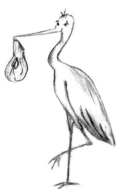

Eating & Delivery

Do not, I repeat, do not eat anything beforehand if you know you're going to be induced, or are having a planned birth or cesarean. Your doctor will tell you this, but just in case you're tempted—don't. The epidural or spinal block may cause you to be nauseated and if you have anything in your stomach, you could end up vomiting throughout labor and delivery!

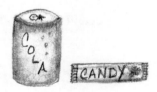

Inductions

If your doctor wants to induce you, you may have the option to check in to the hospital the night before instead of early in the morning. Does anyone function well at 5:00 a.m.?

Pitocin is a synthetic hormone, which is often used to induce labor. Be sure to read the pros and cons of using Pitocin in order to induce. If the Pitocin is not administered at the proper time, it can cause a very long (and more painful) labor. Inducing too soon can also compromise Baby's health. Be sure to consider the option of induction very carefully.

The Natural Birth ...

Sure, what could be more natural than having to push a seven-pound watermelon out what is now (at its best) a one-inch hole? I'm not sure why the vaginal birthing process is the way it is. A question best left to the Man upstairs. The good thing is that God has also equipped some of us with brilliant minds bursting with fantastic inventions like the epidural! But the decision to use drugs during labor is a personal choice. Read about the benefits (if not obvious) and the risks and decide for yourself if you think you can push that seven-pound watermelon through your one-inch hole without pain medicine...hmmm.

There are three stages of labor: Stage One is the pre-labor and dilation phase and can last anywhere from 10 to 12 hours for a woman who has not given birth before. Stage Two is the birthing process and lasts between 1 and 2 hours, and Stage Three is the post birthing process where the placenta and membranes are expulsed after the birth of Baby. This stage only lasts about 15 to 20 minutes. However, there are really no normal timelines for the labor process. Every woman is different and may experience different things throughout each of these phases but there are general things that you can expect.

Dilation means that your cervix is beginning to open in preparation for childbirth. It is measured in centimeters or "fingers" to be less exact. Most people do not feel strong contractions until they are dilated to around four centimeters. Once you are "fully dilated," your cervix is dilated to 10 centimeters and you are ready to give birth.

If you choose to have an epidural, the anesthesiologist will not usually administer the epidural until you are dilated to a four or five, as it slows down labor.

pixie dust

The epidural can wear off. If you begin to feel pain, let the nurses know immediately so that another epidural may be administered.

Suction or forceps may be used to help Baby along. Discuss these methods with your doctor beforehand to find out which will be used and under what circumstances the use of these instruments might be necessary.

Your one-inch hole may quickly become three or four inches ... therefore you may have to have an episiotomy (the doctor will cut the perineum, so you don't tear). If you have an episiotomy or if you tear, you will have to have stitches so that you heal properly.

Perineal massages can be performed to help avoid episiotomies. A perineal massage is when your doctor or labor nurse massages the tissue between the vagina and the anus. It is intended to "stretch" the skin so that an episiotomy is not necessary. It doesn't always work and often times an episiotomy or stitches are needed anyway due to tearing. Supposedly, it is not a comfortable experience. My thoughts ... why risk having to go through more uncomfortable steps that aren't absolutely necessary when it might not even work? Again, you've got enough going on!

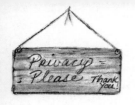

After Birth?

By this time so many people have seen you naked, you're probably wondering if there's a YouTube video of you out there somewhere on the Internet. But if it still matters to you that your ever so slightly swollen and stretched areas are exposed for all the world to see, then be sure to let your doctors and nurses know what your intent is regarding visitors immediately after birth. Some doctors will let everyone who's anyone in the room before they've even completed your stitches. And, if you decide to breastfeed, you may want to nurse Baby right away and you may want this to be a private time as well.

The best way to ensure that outsiders are aware of your intentions is to make a sweet note and have someone post it on the door. Your note could say something like "Private time. Thank you for allowing parents and Baby private bonding time. We appreciate you and will invite you in to see us shortly!"

C-Sections:
Short for Cesarean Sections

(Read Just In Case)

"It won't happen to me..." Did you know, according to the National Center for Health Statistics, that one out of three babies is delivered via unplanned c-section? You may not think you need this information, but do yourself (and your baby) a favor. Read it. Learn about c-section births from the Internet, take a class if your hospital offers it, and talk with friends who have had cesareans. Learn why doctors decide to go this route and what happens during the operation, immediately afterwards, and about the recovery. The more prepared you are, the better off you will be!

C-Section = Childbirth − Pain

(for the most part!)

Someone once said "every cloud has a silver lining," so let's see, what are the positives to c-sections? You get to have a baby and not experience the pain of labor (usually!). You don't have to worry about your vaginal muscles being stretched from here to kingdom come. You don't have to worry about episiotomies. You don't have to remember Lamaze or breathing techniques or finding your "happy place." Your vagina won't hurt after a c-section (other parts will for a while, but we aren't talking about that right now!). You get to know exactly when your baby will be born—give or take a few minutes—no long, drawn-out labor process. And you get to stay in the hospital just a little longer!

The flip side of c-sections? Well, a quick rundown would go something like this: it is major surgery, meaning your body will be opened up, organs moved around, abdominal muscles cut in half, larger epidural needles, possible nausea and severe shaking from the anesthesia, a risk of uterine infection, a risk of Baby not expelling amniotic fluid from lungs properly, and there will be a longer recovery period than one would have with a vaginal delivery.

Now that you are scared out of your wits, please know that most c-sections go very smoothly and you will be so full of excitement for the birth of your baby that you will barely have time to blink over what's happening. But, not knowing what to expect can make it a little scary. This section provides a little more detail on the basic occurrences before, during, and after a c-section. *Please* read on ...

Emergency C-Sections

12:00 p.m.: big lunch—you are, after all, eating for two. 3:00 p.m.: snack. 5:00 p.m.: you feel funny, so you run up to the hospital to have the nurses check you "just to be safe." 6:00 p.m.: you're in labor and you have to have a c-section as soon as possible! Your anesthesiologist is fighting with your doctor, demanding that the c-section wait at least eight hours after you've eaten but extreme circumstances will often prevail and you'll have to go in earlier. Risks? If your food isn't digested, you could vomit and aspirate that vomit into your lungs. But, it doesn't happen very often. If you know anesthesia makes you nauseated—tell them! They can give you something beforehand to help prevent it!

The Procedure

Have you ever watched the television sitcom Scrubs? Scrubs centers around hospital situations which might give us normal laymen (or women) some insight as to how our doctors and nurses deal with what might seem to be life threatening and scary to us, yet are just another daily occurrence to them. Despite the seriousness of all that seems to be going on in your mind...your doctors and nurses do this every day. If you could see it from their eyes, you might find all that happens in a "day in the life of your Labor and Delivery Nurse" to be quite comical. Especially with descriptions that go something like this:

Cold: the sub-zero liquid used to sterilize your pubic area just after they shave you bald.

A Catha-whater? (Catheter): That strange thing hanging out of your nether region used to catch fluids (yes, pee) during and after the procedure.

OR: Operating Room, also known as "Antarctica" as it is just slightly below freezing in here. This is where they will take you to have your baby. Piles of heated blankets may be placed on top of you … *ask for more.*

Spinal Block: Not a football term though you can imagine little guys blocking your pain receptors for you—bless their little pointed heads! Yes, there is a needle, yes, it is long, yes, it hurts—but only for a minute! An anesthesiologist will administer the spinal anesthesia or spinal epidural into an area just below the spinal column using a needle, which will numb the lower half of the body. Both techniques are commonly referred to as spinal blocks though all three terms are slightly different. These techniques have about the same effect but the spinal epidural is a continuous drip of anesthesia. This allows for a little more flexibility during the cesarean (and for pain management after) whereas the spinal anesthesia is administered once and usually lasts throughout the duration of the cesarean. Once you've been given your spinal anesthesia, the rest is cake … mmmm … cake!

pixie dust

Spouse or Coach has to wait outside until after the spinal block, they can then come back in to hold your hand (they won't be doing much else!).

No, you cannot go to jail for pre-birth "shaken baby syndrome." You might wonder this as your body is violently shaking just after they've administered the spinal block. Some do, some don't. Just know that shaking is normal (and unfortunately so is the nausea) and both will subside within a few hours. If the nausea doesn't, your nurse can give you a little "cocktail" to make it go away!

Remember the tingling or numbing sensation you get when your foot is asleep? This is similar to what the lower half of your body will feel like as those little anesthesia guys with pointed heads rush to their places to protect you from feeling what's happening to your body. Certain unknown instruments will be drug across your body at various places to determine whether or not these little guys are doing their jobs. If they are, oh let the fun begin!

Welcome to ... the Twilight Zone: The curtain is up; you can't see a thing. You feel pressure and a bunch of jostling around. The radio is on, and your nurses and doctors are singing along to "It's a Beautiful Morning!" or "Brown-Eyed Girl" all the while holding the life of your unborn child in their hands. You look up and over the curtain at your doctor to see what you thought was a clown face laughing at you, and maybe that really was a gorilla that just walked into the room. You're still shaking and you're beginning to wonder if you're having just another crazy pregnancy dream when you hear ... a tiny cry. There is no other sound in the world except for this cry. All the emotions you've had throughout the pregnancy and during the birth culminate into one *giant* sob, and your new little one is pressed against you, this face you've waited so long to see says, "I know you ... " and all is well with the world.

It's a 10! No, this is not your score for your performance during your c-section, nor is it the length of your baby's genitalia during measurements (though that would be cause for celebration ... but only if it's a boy!). This is what is known as the APGAR score (Appearance, Pulse, Grimace, Activity, Respiration) and is the score of your baby's overall health. 10 being the best ... 7 and above are normal. Baby will usually receive an APGAR score whether you've delivered via c-section or vaginal delivery.

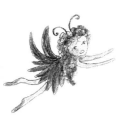

NICU Babies

NICU! Bless you! This is the Natal Intensive Care Unit. Sometimes babies who are delivered via c-section are unable to expel the fluids from their lungs (since they aren't being forced down the birth canal) and this can cause breathing difficulties. Baby may need to spend some time on a respirator, usually to be taken off within hours after birth.

All joking aside, here are a few serious notes on NICU Babies. There is fear in the unknown, and while we don't like to focus on anything negative, it's good to know a few things should Baby have to spend some time in the NICU.

If you have a cesarean and Baby has to go to the NICU, you may be unable to see Baby until you can get up and into a wheelchair to be taken to the NICU, which also means you may not be able to nurse right away. However, a lactation nurse will help you begin the pumping process and you will at least be able to provide the NICU with your colostrum and milk once Baby is ready to eat (usually 36 to 48 hours).

When you go to the NICU, be prepared for tight security and extreme cleanliness. You will be asked to scrub before entering. Usually, no one can be admitted without Baby's parent or special instructions relating otherwise.

Learn the machines and what they do. Take paper and pen to write things down; you'll be so involved with Baby you won't remember a word that's said.

Baby may have to spend some time under "the lights" for jaundice. This is called phototherapy and assists in the removal of bilirubin (produced from the breakdown of red blood cells) from the blood. Sometimes the liver is not mature enough to remove the bilirubin from the blood.

pixie dust

You can call the NICU any time to check on Baby's status—even in the middle of the night. The nurses will always be glad to hear from you!

Ask the NICU nurses about Kangarooing: Your bare skin to Baby's bare skin. This promotes attachment and healing. Kangarooing has been proven to regulate breathing and increase oxygen—both are very good if Baby has had to spend time on a respirator. But most importantly, baby needs you close.

It's difficult to spend nine months with a child growing inside you and then give birth only to come home knowing Baby is still at the hospital. You may experience separation anxiety. If you experience this, and think you might not be able to handle it, your doctor can give you something to help you sleep and can also prescribe something for anxiety.

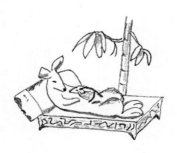

Back to After Birth ...

If you're adamant about nursing Baby right away, be sure to notify the nurses beforehand. If Baby is in good health, they won't deny you, but if Baby needs a little extra attention, you'll have to wait.

pixie dust

You can send Baby to the nursery if you need some rest. If you want to send Baby to the nursery at night, the nursery nurses will wake you for feedings—just be sure to ask!

"WAH ... WAH-WAH ... WAH?" Yes, Charlie Brown, this is exactly what your doctors and nurses say to you after you've had your baby. Well, at least this is what you will hear, and probably all you will remember! Have someone write down what the nurses and doctors say ... you will feel like you're in a dream and will only remember bits and pieces!

pixie dust

Remember to write down the names of doctors and nurses, and visitor's names and gifts (like flowers and who gave them to you—in case the cards get separated). You may want to send a thank you card or basket to your doctors and labor and delivery nurses.

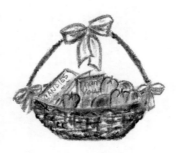

Remember the beer commercial when the guys were so happy about their beer they coined the phrase "I love you Man!"? Well, this is how you will feel as you are all drugged up on pain meds, for the majority of your hospital stay (another added bonus I forgot to mention when discussing the silver lining of c-sections!). Except at 3:00 a.m. when your pain pill has worn off thirty minutes ago and you are beginning to feel the full ramifications of the major surgery you just had. To avoid this, set an alarm clock to go off thirty minutes before you are due for your next pill. Call for your pill, even if you are not in pain, so that the nurses have time to get them to you before the meds wear off. This happens quickly and the pain is very, very sneaky!

pixie dust

Pain meds can make you sick at your stomach. Eat a little bite when you take your meds. Cranberry juice and granola bars or crackers are great!

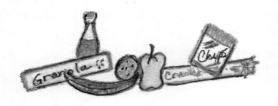

But if, for some reason, you experience a "rude awakening" by the throbbing and aching in your abdomen, ask for hot water pads in addition to your medicine. These really ease the pain and help you relax until your medication kicks in.

That "thing" that's hanging from your nether region, the catheter, will probably be removed the next day. When you get up to go to the bathroom, you may feel a downward flush of um…fluids (okay, blood) when you first stand up. This is normal for both c-sections and vaginal deliveries. When you pee, expect a lot of blood. You will have a *massive* period for several days.

pixie dust

Use the rinse bottles provided by the hospital to help clean up down there. These are squirt bottles that you fill with warm water when you sit to go to the bathroom. Use the warm water to cleanse and soothe the vaginal area. It's kind of weird but it really does help!

Here is the one time in your life where you will fart and want the whole world to know it! You can't leave the hospital until you've passed gas and had a BM (bowel movement). It takes a while for this to happen because your insides have been juggled around and when it does, it can be very painful. Just be prepared!

Okay, Here Comes the Crazy Lady!

First of all, you are not to blame! Any doctor or person who tells you that you just need to "grow up" should be shot on sight! This used to be the general advice provided by doctors back in the day. Now, however, we've wised up and actually learned that there really is something to those chemical imbalances otherwise known as the baby blues or post partum depression.

Don't hesitate to talk with someone about this—it's a normal part of recovery. But if it gets too difficult for you to handle, tell your doctor and make sure your family is aware of the signs of post-partum depression so that they can get you help if you are too far gone to recognize it!

The Days to Come ...

In the days to come, you will feel like you're on a soap opera. You're emotions will be out of whack (happy, sad, happy, sad, happy, sad,) you won't be sure of anything—like what to do with yourself when Baby is sleeping. And you will even catch yourself (as you watch your beautiful, sleeping baby) with a cheesy but wonderful feeling that all really is well with the world. This rather euphoric roller coaster ride of emotions and events will leave you exhausted and sometimes confused as you try to adjust to your wonderful new life with Baby. When the coaster hits a "bottom," it's nice to know what's normal and what might not be normal and what to do if you suspect it's not!

Feelings of detachment from Baby, wondering why you're not instantly in love with your precious one, and scary feelings of inadequacy in regards to whether or not you will actually be a good and protective parent are all normal concerns during the first few months after birth. You may weep with happiness and sometimes sadness for no apparent reason. You may feel helpless, confused, disoriented, and frustrated. All of this is a normal part of recovery and is usually to do with the regulation of hormones within your body.

However, extensive crying, neglect, or dangerous thoughts to yourself or Baby are all signs of post partum depression, which can be a severe psychological disorder if not properly treated. If you or your loved ones notice any of these signs, please seek help from a medical professional immediately!

Home, Sweet Home!

Take it easy! Despite what everyone says, you are not Wonder Woman (unless you are Diana Prince, of course. If you are, skip this... you can do anything!).

For the rest of us... it will be difficult to get up out of bed for several days; just take your time and don't overdo. *Let* your family and friends help you. *Let* them come over and clean, do laundry, and bring dinner. This will be the one time in your adult life—for the rest of your life—when *you* don't have to be the primary caretaker of *everything* in the world! Your alias "Mother Theresa" can wait!

Once you've *recovered* from delivery, you may acquire the nick name "bag lady" or "pack mule" as you tote around Baby with a diaper bag, your purse, maybe a breast pump, and maybe even groceries. But for now, especially if you've had a c-section, it's extremely important that you lift *nothing* heavier than Baby.

Should you decide to tempt fate, beware of what can happen if you overdo. If you've had a cesarean, you could experience any or all of the following: torn muscles in your abdominal area, pulled stitches, or a uterine infection, each can be mistaken for the other. If you've pulled stitches—you will bleed excessively. The other two are often difficult to diagnose and can cause excruciating pain. Torn muscles can take up to six weeks to heal and are very, very painful. If you have a uterine infection, they will prescribe you antibiotics to take care of the infection.

If you thought you were a "bloated toad" during the last few months of your pregnancy, and you've had to have a c-section, just wait until they pump you full of Pitocin to get your uterus to contract back down to normal size! For some of us, this synthetic hormone causes us to retain a lot of water. It may take several weeks before your water "lets down" so just be prepared for "cankles" and "pig feet." In fact, the skin on your feet can stretch so tight, and can be so painful you wish someone would pop you like a balloon. If you're extremely uncomfortable, a doctor can prescribe a diuretic, but it's not recommended if you're breastfeeding.

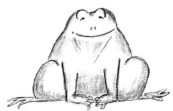

pixie dust

Of all the sleepless nights, recovering from surgery, crying Baby, dirty diapers, and getting Baby to feed, the back pain and muscle pain in general can be a very difficult part of trying to recover. Those muscles just aren't used to all that is now required of them. Backrubs can completely rejuvenate your mind and body! Heating pads and ibuprofen also help!

Hush Little Baby, Don't You Cry!

(Always check with your doctor ...)

Here we are again! It's 3:00 a.m. and Baby just won't be consoled. You feel like you've tried everything—you've changed the diaper, tried to feed, tried to rock and pat to sleep but nothing is working. By this point, Baby's crying is bound to wake the neighbors ... what to do, what to do? Here are a few things to try before calling the doctor in the middle of the night.

First, try gas drops, especially if Baby is drawing up knees and crying. These should be okay to use from day one, but check with your doctor. Gas drops do not interact with other medicines because they do not absorb into Baby's system. If it's gas, this will help to calm Baby almost immediately.

If the gas drops don't work, try Hyland Colic Tablets—more commonly known as the Miracle Medicine! Colic is a diagnosis given when no one seems to know what's really wrong. Babies grow and growing pains hurt, especially when the digestive system is trying to mature. You can dissolve these tablets in water and give to Baby or dissolve directly on the inside of Baby's cheek. Don't hesitate to follow the directions and use them every fifteen minutes until Baby is calm. These are homeopathic and safe to use from day one, but again, check with your doctor.

If the gas drops and the colic tablets don't work, try infant acetaminophen. This will help with pain in general—especially with teething and fevers. But always call the doctor if Baby has a fever. If your doctor makes you feel badly for calling when you're concerned … find another doctor!

Try the four S's: Shooshing, Swaddling, Swinging, and Singing also work to calm a crying baby. Try any combination of these together and one is sure to work!

pixie dust

There are blankets specifically designed for swaddling and are much easier to swaddle with than a regular receiving blanket. Swaddling really helps Baby to feel more secure. Toys and gadgets with heartbeat sounds also help to soothe Baby.

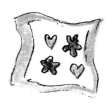

If nothing does the trick and Baby is not running a fever and nothing seems to be out of place on its body (diaper and clothing not binding, fingers and toes all okay), then Baby may just be tired, over stimulated, or just needing to release some tension. If you're a new parent, it can be difficult to decipher what they need when they cry and it's very disheartening when you can't console them, so much to the point that you may cry with them.

pixie dust

Baby's cry signals a hormonal response from your body whether it's your milk letting down or you crying as well. So it's not just you sympathizing or being upset that your baby is crying; it's a physiological reaction.

Cool mist humidifiers can help with stuffy noses (just be sure to wash them once a week!). And baby vapor rub is great to rub on the chest and neck. Just be sure to cover Baby up so little hands don't rub the gel into little eyes.

If Baby really is sick and your doctor has prescribed antibiotics, ask the pharmacy for a syringe (it won't have a needle in it). Have them mark the syringe where to draw up the medicine. Also, ask if it's okay to add water to the medicine or warm it up under hot water. Most antibiotics often have to be kept cold, making them thick, which will make Baby gag and medicine ends up everywhere but in Baby.

pixie dust

Rule of thumb with medicine is that if Baby spits up within five minutes after administering medicine, usually another dose is required, but always ask your doctor or pharmacist to be sure. Many pharmacies are open twenty-four hours so don't hesitate to call!

If Baby wakes up shortly after you lay them down, it's probably because Baby misses your warmth and senses the broken connection. Place a hot water pad in the bed and then be sure to remove the pad just before laying Baby down. Even though they sense the broken connection, they still feel warm and usually go right back to sleep.

Some babies fight sleep and will cry when you try to get them to go to sleep. Usually, you can learn the sleepy cues and avoid the drama but sometimes their frustration, as well as yours, escalates to a point of no return.

Letting Baby "cry it out" is a personal decision that every parent has to make. This is not recommended for babies under six months of age. This is also not recommended for parents who are practicing "attachment" parenting, as it is believed to break trust bonds between child and parent. If this option is something you are considering, please speak with your pediatrician but most importantly … do your research!

Rubber Ducky, You're the One! You Make Bath Time So Much Fun!

Here again, evolution will spring forth your desire to sprout another set of hands. Bath time can be difficult until you get into the swing of things. Here are a few suggestions that will help simplify your bath time routine.

Place everything you will need for bath time in a tote so that you have it all within reach:

- Large and Small Washcloths
- Towels
- Baby Wash
- Scrub Brush
- Baby Oil
- Bath Sling
- Safety Swabs
- Water Toys & Plastic Cup

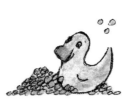

pixie dust

If you're bathing Baby in the kitchen, remember to turn off the air conditioner, so it doesn't blow cold air on Baby while bathing.

Caution: Slippery When Wet!

Babies are surprisingly slippery when wet, so instead of using a baby bath, use a bath sling or foam pad in the kitchen sink for the first several months. Baby just lays on it and you can wash without having to hold the entire body and you don't have to worry about them slipping around in a baby tub. This also helps you to keep from immersing Baby in water until the umbilical cord and/or circumcision has healed.

Jewelry and long nails really tend to get in the way most of the time, especially during bath time. Both can scratch Baby's tender skin...don't make me say "I told you so!"

pixie dust

Place a big, warm, wet washcloth over Baby's belly during bath time. This keeps them warm and makes them feel secure. Remember to rewet it often.

The body is a strange and sometimes smelly organ. Parts like under the arms, neck crevices, ears, and in between fingers and toes like to gather "gunk" and boy, you'll know it soon if you've missed a spot! The stench will make your stomach churn! There are special safety swabs made just for baby ears that will help you clean the wax out without going too far inside the ear. But a thin wash cloth and a little soap and water work just as well.

Contrary to popular belief, cradle cap is not due to unsavory hygiene practices. Some of us are just scared stiff to even touch the "soft spot" on a baby's head much less scrub it during a shampoo! Use a soft scrub brush (or get one from the hospital) to gently scrub Baby's head, including the soft spot, in order to prevent or eliminate cradle cap.

pixie dust

Ever wonder what baby oil was really for? If Baby does get cradle cap, use a little bit of baby oil and scrub it in the affected area. Let it sit while washing Baby, then wash with baby shampoo and scrub gently. You can also use vegetable oil!

It's also nerve wracking to try to clip Baby's nails during the first few months, so use an emery board and file them for now. You'll eventually get the hang of it!

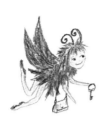

Out and About

Being a new mom comes with special societal "perks." But there are a lot of things you'll have to learn how to do differently with Baby in tow. You begin to morph into what you used to know as your own over-protective mother. You start to think differently and somehow have extraterrestrial senses. Yes, your mother really did have eyes in the back of her head and this is how she got them.

Grocery carts… Most of us, as good Samaritans, try to return our carts to the cart return when we are done. If, however, you were unable to park next to a cart return, you get to leave the cart by your car without feeling guilty.

Beware of Stranger Danger! You'll find there are a lot of things that complete strangers offer to help you with when toting a child (like taking your cart to the cart return for you or helping you with groceries). But just be careful, as this can make you easy prey as well.

pixie dust

Get your keys out before you leave the store. Park near lighted areas and try to stay away from vans or SUVs when parking. Look under your car as you walk toward it to make sure no one is underneath. If you can, get in the back seat and lock the doors while buckling in Baby. Always make sure back car doors are locked when filling up at the gas station. Just be sure to take your keys with you.

Now is the time to begin good habits. From here on out, for the rest of your days as a Mom … always keep antibacterial wipes and tissues with you. Buy antibacterial wipes every time you are at the store to keep in your purse. Keep a set of both wipes and tissues in your car. Wipe down grocery carts, highchairs and tables with wipes. Try to remember to sneeze into your elbow sleeve instead of into your hand (with which you will undoubtedly touch Baby). Remember to wash your hands and use antibacterial sanitizer often.

Flying objects in the car can be dangerous to Baby as well as any plastic bags that might be within their reach. Try to put groceries in the trunk.

Diaper Bag Necessities

With Baby and baby carrier and diaper bag, you'll have a lot on your hands so consolidate and use the diaper bag as your purse!

- Diapers, Wipes, and Ointment
- Changing Pad and Receiving Blankets
- Medicines–Baby's and Yours
- Disposable Diaper Bags
- Bibs, Burp Cloths, and Pacifiers
- Extra Outfits and Socks
- Hat, Comb, Nail File, and Aspirator
- Sunglasses, Pads, and Tissues
- Wallet, Keys, Cell Phone, and Makeup
- Formula if Bottle Feeding
- Bottles, Nipples, and Bottled Water
- Nursing Pads
- Instant Anti-Bacterial Cleaner / Wipes
- Snacks

Always and Never:

Baby Proofing and Other Safety Tips

Baby will be crawling before you know it and things you meant to do may slip your mind until you actually catch a crawling baby rummaging through your cleaning supplies—wondering how much, if any, was really ingested. Read about baby proofing your home online or purchase a baby proofing book, but here are a few of the most important things you need to know:

Always place knives, matches, scissors, and cleaning agents in locked cabinets.

Always keep electrical outlets covered with sturdy covers.

Always make sure all fire/carbon monoxide detection alarms are in proper working order (test batteries frequently).

Keep the number to the Center for Poison Control in your cell phone and on the refrigerator.

Sticky little fingers are always reaching for tempting things just out of their reach! Always put used knives and other dangerous objects on the back of the counter. *Never* leave bottles with hot liquid sitting on the counter without the tops on and *always* make sure that pot and pan handles are positioned toward the back of the stove so Baby can't reach them and so you don't knock them off. Baby can also reach for knives in an open dishwasher.

Never leave Baby unattended around coffee tables, fireplaces, and steps, as they are frequently the cause of serious injuries to babies.

Never allow Baby to sit or stand on an escalator without your careful guidance. Extreme injuries can occur. If possible, hold Baby or use elevators just to be safe.

Never leave your car unattended with Baby inside, not even in front of the house while you just run in to grab something. *Always* take Baby with you—you'll never forgive yourself should something happen.

Make sure that caregivers are aware of all of these precautions. Sometimes caregivers don't have the heart and mind of a protective mother so just be sure.

Love Is All There Is ...

Out of all the little handy tips, the best advice I can give you is to love your sweet baby unconditionally, and to do what feels right and natural in your heart. You have been blessed with the gift of being able to make the world a better place, one child at a time, and oh what a precious gift it is! Take from this book and from others what you will, but heed what is in your heart. You will raise a beautiful, smart, brave, and strong child with Spirit that knows no bounds! Despite all the questions, uncertainties, worries, aches, and pains...at the end of the day, Love is all there is...you'll see.

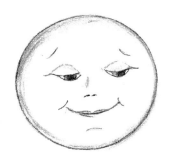

Evening Prayer

Now I lay me down to sleep
I pray the Lord my soul to keep
Love and guard me through the night
And wake me with the morning light.
Amen

Checklist for Purchases

Nursery & Travel Items:

___Crib / Bassinette   ___Sleep Positioner   ___Car Seat

___Travel System   ___Changing Table   ___Pack-n-Play

___Dresser / Baskets ___Bedding / Sheets   ___Monitor

___Diaper Champ   ___Clothes Hamper   ___Rocker

___Swing / Bouncer ___Portable Swing   ___Boppy

___Sling/ Carrier   ___Wipe Warmer   ___Play Mats

___Diapers & Wipes ___Colic Tablets   ___Gas Drops

___Teething Gel   ___Diaper Pail (outside)

___Infant Pain Reliever

Clothing Items:

___Going Home Outfit

___Onsies   ___Gowns   ___Pants

___Socks   ___Bibs   ___Hats

___Detergent   ___Stain Remover   ___Hangers

Bottle Feeding Items:

___Bottles   ___Bottle Warmer   ___Nipples

___Bottle Brushes   ___Burp Cloths   ___Formula

___Formula Holder   ___Liners (optional)

___Bottled Water   ___Dishwasher Baskets

Breast Feeding Items:

___Pump & Accessories	___Nipple Cream	___Milk Bags
___Nipple Shields	___Nursing Bras	___Nursing Pads

Bath Items:

___Bath Sling	___Baby Tub	___Wash Cloths
___Water Toys / Ducky	___Baby Wash	___Baby Oil
___Baby Shampoo	___Baby Lotion	___Towels
___Safety Swabs	___Soft Scrub Brush	___Tote

Diaper Bag Items:

___Wipe Holder	___Diapers	___Wipes
___Receiving Blankets	___Nasal Aspirator	___Pacifiers
___Anti-bacterial Wipes	___Medicines	___Nail File
___Disposable Diaper Bags	___Diaper Rash Ointment	

Necessities for Mommy:

___Toiletries & Makeup	___Girdle Panties	___Camera (etc)
___Going Home Outfit	___Robe & Gown	___Journal
___Ibuprofen	___Heating Pad	___Pedicure
___Batteries	___Pens	___Labor Music / Player

listen|imagine|view|experience

AUDIO BOOK DOWNLOAD INCLUDED WITH THIS BOOK!

In your hands you hold a complete digital entertainment package. Besides purchasing the paper version of this book, this book includes a free download of the audio version of this book. Simply use the code listed below when visiting our website. Once downloaded to your computer, you can listen to the book through your computer's speakers, burn it to an audio CD or save the file to your portable music device (such as Apple's popular iPod) and listen on the go!

How to get your free audio book digital download:

1. Visit www.tatepublishing.com and click on the e|LIVE logo on the home page.
2. Enter the following coupon code:
   767f-a68c-0a75-7646-4877-e653-286d-a31b
3. Download the audio book from your e|LIVE digital locker and begin enjoying your new digital entertainment package today!